Table of Contents

LIST OF WORKSHEETS AND ACTIVITIES
COMPLETED: Write and Date

CHAPTER	Name and Date Completed	PAGE

DEDICATIONS

To all of the individuals who have worked so diligently at improving their

lifestyle and even saving their own lives and who had the courage to ask for and

accept guidance through a rough yet healing journey. Keep up the healthy, self-

care!

CHAPTER 1

Lose Weight Now!

Let's cut to the chase! This book is not about lectures. It is simply about finding out what will work for you to lose weight, and stay that way- healthy! Feel free to skip around this book or read and do the simple, easy-to-follow activities in order. It is up to you. The key is discovering what works. We offer many different types of therapeutic approaches to help with weightloss.

Everyone knows that carrying excess weight doesn't make us feel good, if it were as simple as knowing this fact, I am sure you would not be reading this right now. With that said, we don't need to tell you how hard it can be to successfully lose weight and keep it off. Trying to lose weight can be frustrating and overwhelming. However, if you really want to you will. We would like to offer you genuine hope based on real results. Also, I want you to know that it is not too late to start today. Now is the time to be healthy, attractive & lean. Imagine how nice it is going to feel to lose weight.

Once you decide to have an ideal weight and shape, it happens! You may want to work with a therapist but this may not be needed for success. It can be helpful to have a therapist who holds you accountable for taking the steps to achieve your goals, and checking in with a therapist each week can be very helpful and can help guide you when situations or circumstances arise. You decide.

It can be very frustrating to work on your issues without the guidance and helpful insight of a trained professional. We have included in the back of the book, criteria for helping you choose the right therapist for you. Fortunately, with this guide you will be able to make progress much, much quicker and you will have a handy resource to review if questions or concerns happen to arise during the therapeutic process and in the future.

Remember, throughout your entire life you always move in the general direction of your most dominant thought. So if you keep saying "'I find it difficult to lose weight, if I do I will probably become irritable, and put the weight back on". Then you probably will! If you say instead, "'I am an ideal weight and shape and will be for ever and ever", positive thinking, then the results will be much more effective. You can effectively create your own weightless future!

WEIGHT LOSS QUESTIONNAIRE

This questionnaire is designed to be filled in by clients before commencing first session. You can then use the information gathered during the session.

Your responses to the following questions will enable your therapist to construct and effective program to help you to lose the weight that you want. All information is private and confidential.

How much (approximately) do you weigh?

What is your goal weight?

When in your life were you your ideal weight?

What changed in your life when you began to gain weight?

What emotions do you associate with this period in your life? i.e. guilt, comfort, punishment, contentment, etc.

On an average day, what do you eat and how much?

a) For breakfast

b) Mid-morning

c) Lunch

d) Mid-afternoon

e) Evening meal

f) Supper

g) Other

Do you snack between meals? If so, which meal, and what do you snack on?

Do you ever get up during the night for something to eat?

If you overeat, which of the above foods would you like to cut down on, or cut out altogether?

Approximately how many drinks do you have a day?

Do you drink fizzy or sweetened drinks? If so, how many?

Do you drink alcohol? If so, how many units per day? Per week?

Do you drink water? If so, how many glasses approximately per day?

Who does the food shopping in your household?

Who prepares and cooks the food?

Do you often leave food on your plate?

Do you finish off other people's food?

Do you enjoy: (make a check where appropriate)

Sweet foods?

Savory foods?

Fresh fruit?

Fresh vegetables?

Starchy foods?

Fatty foods?

What suggestions do you feel would be most effective for helping you to achieve your goal weight? (Make a check where appropriate)

Stop overeating

Stop snacking between meals

Stop drinking alcohol

Stop drinking sweet drinks

Stop eating junk foods

Take more exercise

Have more energy

Other

Are, or were, either of your parents, brothers or sisters overweight? If so, please say which.

Do you remember any instances of being 'forced' to eat up when you were younger? YES / NO

Was food ever used as a reward for doing something good? YES / NO

Did you ever eat to forget about something else? YES / NO

Did you often feel hungry as a child? YES / NO

Do you ever eat when you are not hungry? YES / NO
If yes, please give an example.

Do you ever eat to please someone else? YES / NO
If yes, please give an example.

Are you constantly thinking about the next meal? YES / NO

Do you have any problematic relationships in your life at present YES / NO
If yes, please state with whom.

If you answered yes, how do you see this relationship improving?

How many hours sleep (approximately) do you have per night?

Exercise

Do you lead an active life? YES / NO

Does your job involve sitting down a lot? YES / NO

Are you involved in any sport or regular exercise YES / NO

If the answer to the above question is no, can you identify a sport that you would enjoy doing? YES / NO

If yes, please say what this would be

When would a convenient time for you to do this, be?

List Medications

Are you currently taking any drugs or prescribed medication? YES / NO

If yes, are you aware of any side effects from these that could cause weight gain YES / NO

If yes, are you willing to consult with your GP to find a more suitable alternative YES / NO.

WHY LOSE WEIGHT?

Know your reasons why you want to lose weight. List the reasons.

1.

2.

3.

4.

5.

6.

7.

8.

9.

10.

FOOD AND REWARDS

Now that you are aware of why you want to lose weight, let's look at the benefits that you mistakenly believe that you gain from your current eating habits. List them here.

Taking breaks at work or during chores.
A "reward" after completing a task.
Comfort
A quick get away
Relieve boredom
Social Aspects

Challenge: Are these reasons just excuses? Are they just perceived benefits? What are some positive activities you could replace your current eating habits with? For example, you don't need to have food for comfort. Take a bath or call a friend instead. Enjoy an ice cold, refreshing glass of water.

THE BENEFITS OF BEING A HEALTHY WEIGHT

What are the benefits that you will enjoy about losing weight?

How much more self confident will you be?

How proud will you, your friends, and family be?

How will your role as a healthy person impact your children?

How will your health improve? Energy…

FOCUS ON YOUR STRENGTHS

List reasons why and how you can and will lose weight.

1.

2.

3.

4.

5.

6.

7.

8.

9.

10.

ANTICIPATING OBSTACLES

What are some potential triggers that you may anticipate that could interfere with your goal of losing weight?

1.

2.

3.

4.

5.

6.

7.

8.

9.

10.

LET'S MAKE IT AS EASY AS POSSIBLE FOR YOU TO QUIT

Look at your list of potential triggers and let's plan to make this as painless as possible for you. Write down the trigger and the possible solution to the problem.

Suggestions:
Do some spring cleaning in your kitchen cabinets
Clean out your fridge.
Let others know about your goal of losing weight.
Remove the temptations.
Alter your routine.
Throw away reminders such as junk food and candy.

ADVERTISE IT

Advertise that you have decided to lose weight. Let everyone know your goal. Keeping your goal your own little secret may make it easier to give in. It is important to lose weight for yourself but it can't hurt to have the encouragement and support form friends and loved ones. Involving others may help motivate you to achieve your goal.

This is a big deal! Let others share in on your progress and success. Who knows you may become a positive role model for others who may get inspired by your efforts and success.

Call friends
Email family
Write letters
Send out announcements
Plan a celebration

Make a list of who you will involve:

GO ON AND REWARD YOURSELF

If you graduated from college, got a promotion, or succeeded in some way, chances are, you would celebrate your accomplishment! You have worked hard, earned success, and deserve to treat yourself. Losing weight is a huge accomplishment so go on and reward yourself. I would like for you to actually mark some dates on your calendar to recognize your achievement and positive change that you have made in your life. Maybe for a two-week milestone, you choose to reward yourself with a new outfit. At the end of the year you may choose to take a vacation. You choose!

Write down your planned rewards:

Pat yourself on the back. Well-Done!

LOOK AT THE IMPACT AND CONSEQUENCES

Imagine in great detail the impact of unhealthy eating. What does this impact look like? Be specific.

How has your eating habits affected the way you look or may look in the future?

Notice the affect on your skin, the increase in blemishes.

How do you feel about your children and significant other living through terminal illness with you?

What will the long-term impact of unhealthy eating habits be on your children as they watch you grow bigger and bigger?

A NEW CHAPTER

We want you to recognize that you are now heading in a different direction and leaving unhealthy eating habits behind. Unhealthy eating was once a bad habit that you have overcome and food does not define who you are. You will no longer label yourself "fat". Focus on what this feels like for you.

Any fears? Are you excited? Nervous? Ready?

Write the title of your new chapter and a summary of what your story is all about.

BEING FAT SUCKS!

Think about a time when you wished that you were thinner. Maybe when you were at your daughter's dance recital and a little girl pointed at you because you were over weight. Or when you were out of breath walking up a short flight of stairs.

Write these negative memories down.

Now, I would like for you to play these memories in your head like you were watching a movie. Replay them vividly. Emphasize the negativity. See how this negativity strengthens your decision to lose weight.

CHAPTER 2

Self-Soothe, Distract, & Relax!

SELF-SOOTHE & DISTRACT

You can regulate the way that you think and feel by using self-soothing and distraction techniques.

Self-soothing techniques can be used to calm yourself down and relax when you are upset. The goal of self-soothing skills is to comfort yourself when you experience distress such as experiencing symptoms associated with unhealthy eating habits. By doing things that are sensually pleasant and, most especially, not harmful, you can overcome negative thoughts and feelings.

Distraction techniques can be effective in helping reduce the anxiety, urges, withdrawal symptoms, and cravings associated with eating in an unhealthy manner. These techniques do just what the name implies. They distract you from unhealthy eating habits. Instead of engaging in an unhealthy activity like eating junk food, you replace it with a healthy, positive activity that will help you take your mind off of food and you focus on the activity at hand.

SELF-SOOTHING TECHNIQUES

Formulate a self-soothing plan to use when you have the urge to eat unhealthy foods. Be sure to make lists for use at home, at work, and when you are away from home. You may recognize that these soothing techniques are activities that you already engage in. Others may have never thought of the activities this way. Learning how to self soothe is simply learning how to make yourself feel better. Therefore, alleviate negative thoughts, feelings, and emotions. Be creative, just writing ideas is a distraction technique.

Here are some ideas using your five senses:

Taste (use with caution)

Smell

Vision

Hearing

Touch

Make check marks next to the items on the following pages that you could potentially use. Add your own self-soothing techniques to each list. Keep these lists handy for future reference.

EATING MEDITATION

You eat every day, but how often do you really pay attention to what you are eating while you are eating it? Do you usually eat with other people? In front of the TV? While reading? Can you usually finish a three course meal in ten minutes or less?

The following is a conscious eating meditation. In the beginning, try it someplace where it is unlikely anyone will come over and eat with you. As you practice this conscious eating meditation you may begin to implement this awareness within your daily meals and snack with others.

1. Sit down in front of your food and take several deep breaths. Note the color, shape, and texture. Does it seem appealing to you? Can you barely restrain yourself from immediately consuming this food? Whatever you are feeling, NOTICE it.

2. Be aware of your intentions to begin eating. Is this a food that you want to ingest into your body? Just simply notice your feelings about what you are about to eat. Move your hand slowly toward the food. As you do this, make a quiet mental note of the action. You may say to yourself, "reaching…..reaching…..reaching." by labeling your action you are more likely to keep in mind your purpose- to stay AWARE. As you pick up the food, notice that you are lifting…..lifting…..lifting.

3. Watch your hand move the food closer to your mouth. When it nears your mouth, take a moment to smell the food. What smells do you recognize? How is your body reacting to the smells? Is your mouth watering? Notice the sensation of your body desiring food.

4. As you take your first bite, feel your teeth penetrate the food. When the bite is complete, how is the food positioned in your mouth? How does your tongue position the food so that it is between your teeth? Begin chewing slowly. What are the sensations in your teeth? Your tongue? How does your tongue move when you chew? What tastes are you experiencing? What part of your tongue experiences the taste? Where is your arm? Did you put it back on the table? If so, did you notice the motion?

5. When you swallow the food, try to be aware of how the muscles in your esophagus contract and relax as they push the food to your stomach. What size is it? Is it empty, full, or somewhere in between?

6. As you continue to eat, try to stay aware of as many sensations as you can. Silently label each movement if this helps. Try eating with the hand you don't normally use, because the awkwardness may serve as a reminder to pay attention. As with your basic meditation, when thoughts arise, notice them and then return your attention to your food.

SELF-SOOTHING

TASTE

- ☐ Take advantage of your recuperating taste buds and have a healthy low calorie treat.

- ☐ Eat slowly and savor every bite.

- ☐ Cook a favorite low calorie meal.

- ☐ Drink a soothing drink low in calories like Herbal tea.

- ☐ Drink ice cold, crisp water.

- ☐ Practice an eating meditation.

- ☐ Notice the texture of food and drinks on your tongue.

- ☐ Eat a sugar free Popsicle.

- ☐ Suck on a piece of sugar free candy.

- ☐ Chew gum.

- ☐ Create a means of enjoying foods that help you and do not cause weight gain.

- ☐
- ☐
- ☐

SELF-SOOTHING

SMELL

☐ Smell breakfast, lunch, or dinner being cooked at home or in a restaurant.

☐ Take a walk in a garden and smell the flowers.

☐ Take a hike in the woods and smell the trees and foliage.

☐ Go outside just after it rains.

☐ Breath in the smells of nature.

☐ Light a scented candle.

☐ Burn incense.

☐ Try new low-calorie recipes and take in all of the yummy and healthy smells.

☐ Put on perfume.

☐ Keep a significant other's perfume on a piece of cloth or book-mark with you so that you feel a sense of being with this comforting person.

☐

☐

☐

☐

☐

SELF-SOOTHING

VISION

☐   Take a walk in a pretty part of town.

☐   Look at nature around you.

☐   Buy some flowers and put them where you can see them.

☐   Go to an art museum.

☐   Sit in a beautiful garden and enjoy the scenery.

☐   Look at old photos.

☐   Watch the rain or snow fall.

☐   Watch the flames of a candle burning.

☐   Read a "coffee table" picture book.

☐   Watch a movie.

☐   Read a book.

☐   Get your nails done so they look pretty.

☐   Watch birds soaring in the sky.

☐   Make animals and shapes out of clouds.

☐   Look at the stars and moon in the night's sky.

☐   Go to a performing arts show.

☐

SELF-SOOTHING

HEARING

- ☐ Listen to different types of music.

- ☐ Notice how different kinds of music makes you feel.

- ☐ Listen to nature.

- ☐ Listen to a tape of nature or to the sounds of the ocean.

- ☐ Sit by a waterfall or fountain.

- ☐ Be mindful and let the sounds be the center of your attention.

- ☐ Learn how to play a musical instrument.

- ☐

- ☐

- ☐

- ☐

- ☐

- ☐

SELF-SOOTHING

TOUCH

- ☐ Take a bubble bath.

- ☐ Pet your dog or cat.

- ☐ Snuggle with a baby.

- ☐ Get cozy in blankets.

- ☐ Put lotion on.

- ☐ Float in a pool.

- ☐ Go swimming.

- ☐ Walk barefoot on fresh cut grass.

- ☐ Get a massage.

- ☐ Experience whatever it is that you are touching.

- ☐ Put clean sheets on your bed.

- ☐ Put a cold or hot compress on a body part.

- ☐ Hug someone.

- ☐ Brush your hair.

- ☐ Floss and brush your teeth.

- ☐

- ☐

YOUR SELF-SOOTHING PLAN

☐

☐

☐

☐

☐

☐

☐

☐

☐

☐

☐

DISTRACTION TECHNIQUES

Formulate a distraction plan to use when you have the urge to eat unhealthy food. Be sure to make lists for use at home, at work, and when you are away from home. Like the self-soothing techniques, you may recognize that these distraction techniques are activities that

you already engage in. However, others may have never thought of theses distracting activities this way.

Here is a list of ideas to use as distraction techniques:

Make check marks next to the items on the following pages that you could potentially use. Be sure to add your own techniques to the list so that when you need them they are right where you wrote them.

DISTRACT YOURSELF

DISTRACT YOURSELF WITH ACTIVITIES:

☐ Exercise

☐ Go for a walk

☐ Go Hiking

☐ Go to the movies

☐ Sew or knit

☐ Participate in sports

☐ Do the dishes

☐ Clean the house

☐ Gardening

☐ Engage in hobbies of interest

☐ Go fishing

☐ Swimming

☐ Painting

☐ Journaling

☐ Scrap-booking

☐ Arts and crafts

☐ Rearrange a room

- ☐ Organize drawers or closets

- ☐ Clean your car

- ☐ Take a dog for a walk

- ☐ Go to the park

- ☐ Take a class of interest

- ☐ Research a topic on the internet.

- ☐ Catch up on work

- ☐ Call a friend or family member

- ☐ Read

- ☐ Put a puzzle together

- ☐ Complete a crossword puzzle

- ☐ Play a game

- ☐ Go window-shopping

- ☐ Daydream

- ☐ Go to church

- ☐ Attend a support group

- ☐ Meditate

- ☐ Practice yoga

- ☐ Join a gym

- ☐ Fix something that may be broken.

DISTRACT YOURSELF BY FOCUSING ON

OTHERS:

☐   Volunteer

☐   Care for a family member in need

☐   Help a neighbor

☐   Give something to someone else

☐   Do something nice for someone

☐   Give your significant other a massage

☐   Plan a surprise for someone

☐   Play with a child

☐   Help someone clean their car or house

☐   Write someone a letter

☐   Send an email.

☐

☐

☐

☐

☐

YOUR DISTRACTION PLAN

☐

☐

☐

☐

☐

☐

☐

☐

☐

☐

☐

CHAPTER 3

Self-Hypnosis

First, let's go ahead and release all of those misconceptions and misunderstandings about hypnosis that may have been acquired throughout the years. Many individuals may be apprehensive about hypnotic techniques due to the lack of knowledge and understanding of the therapeutic advantages of hypnosis. Here are the facts about hypnosis, plain and simple.

What hypnosis is NOT:

∅ Hypnosis is not mind control.

∅ Hypnosis is not magic nor faith healing. Although, it helps if the client has confidence in the practitioner and faith in his or her own ability to heal.

∅ Hypnosis is not sleep nor does one loose consciousness.

∅ Hypnosis cannot make you do or say anything that you would not normally do or say.

∅ Hypnosis does not weaken your will power. It actually strengthens it.

What hypnosis IS:

⊕ Hypnosis is the ability to achieve desired goals by completely focusing.

⊕ All Hypnosis is self-hypnosis.

⊕ Hypnosis is deep relaxation with an acute sense of awareness.

⊕ Hypnosis is similar to meditation and dream states.

⊕ Hypnosis utilizes the power of positive suggestion and thinking. Anyone can reject a suggestion if it does not correspond with their belief systems.

⊕ Anyone is capable of hypnosis.

⊕ It is believed that the more intelligent one is, the easier they may be hypnotized.

⊕ Hypnosis allows clients to use their own minds to make desired changes.

Just as medicine combines both art and science, so does hypnotherapy. After a session of hypnotherapy clients may feel profound relaxation and peace. Hypnosis is a feeling that must be experience to fully appreciate.

Hypnosis has evolved into a well-respected practice and today it is used by certified hypnotherapists, doctors, psychologists, psychotherapists, and law enforcement professionals. This technique is utilized in a variety of ways, for instance, pain management, stress-related disorders, anesthesia, psychotherapy and memory recall. It is also used as a tool to help manage a wide range of phobic, anxiety and other psychological disorders.

Hypnotherapy is completely safe and helpful. It is a natural state of mind.

Hypnosis is a method of changing your thoughts, behaviors, and even your body... Using the power of your mind!

Hypnosis works by guiding you into a deep state of relaxation. During this stage of relaxation, the hypnotherapist (or hypnosis recording) begins providing the subconscious mind with positive suggestions and stories to help achieve the goals of the individual.

Hypnosis is one of the quickest and most exciting ways to make positive, lasting change in your life.

Hypnosis works by guiding the mind into a state of deep relaxation. In this "trance" state, the critical filtering capabilities of the conscious mind are bypassed, allowing the hypnotherapist to provide suggestions direct to the subconscious mind... the "control panel" of the brain.

Hypnosis also works by the hypnotherapist talking in the "language" of the subconscious mind, ensuring the conscious mind doesn't interfere at all. This is achieved through a combination of guided visualization exercises and through the use of Neuro Linguistic Programming (NLP).

Studies have shown that intelligent people are actually easier to hypnotize. And it doesn't matter if you're skeptical of the process... the fact you're trying hypnosis shows you have an open mind. The results will prove themselves!

Hypnosis is a soothing state similar to the state we enter before falling asleep. Everyone probably has already experienced hypnosis, for example; when you were driving and many, many minutes have gone by and you were off daydreaming yet you managed to safely arrive at your destination, or you are reading a book or watching a movie and you are fully lost in it, perhaps showing emotion.

Hypnosis is a totally natural and completely safe method of self-development... and can help you achieve goals you never thought possible! You will be able to lose weight now!

Self-hypnosis scripts will assist you in weight loss.

It is important that you read these scripts daily. Preferably, read the scripts in the morning before starting your day, at noon or in the middle of your day, and in the evening before going to sleep. Also, self-hypnosis can be used as a tool as needed when you crave or have an urge to eat.

You may choose to read the scripts or tape record your voice reading the scripts. You choose. A recording can be powerful yet reading can be more convenient at times. You may also choose to do a combination of both.

PREPARE FOR SELF-HYPNOSIS

Before reading the script, get comfortable either sitting up or lying down. Take some deep breaths. Inhale and exhale with ease. Your exhale is twice as long as your inhale. Allow yourself to relax. Focus on your breathing. Fill your lungs with clean fresh air and when you exhale release all the air out of your lungs. Letting go and releasing any tension or anxiety that you may be holding. As you allow yourself to relax even more now. Sense the beating of your own heart. Use the power of your mind to slow that heartbeat down. Just a bit, just seeing whether you can use the power of your mind to slow that heartbeat down just a little. So that you can then feel your whole body slowing down... becoming lazier and heavier because you have nothing else to do here except relax and read. Focus on the words. Use your imagination. You have nothing whatsoever to do except to relax now. You have set this time for self care. Nobody wanting anything, nobody is expecting anything... so you can allow your whole body to continue to relax. Know that you are taking care of yourself now. Right here, right now. Release any tension. Relax your jaws, your neck, shoulders. Allow your tongue to just rest in your mouth. Be sure it is not pressed against the roof of your mouth. Relax your arms, abdomen, legs and feet. Completely relaxed from the top of your head to the tip of your toes. When you are ready you may begin self-hypnosis.

SELF-HYPNOSIS SCRIPTS

SELF-HYPNOSIS SCRIPTS FOR WEIGHT REDUCTION I, II, III

Weight Reduction I

Weight Reduction Session I

You have begun a positive approach to obtain the slim, healthy, attractive body, which you desire. I am going to give you some suggestions that will make this a permanent change in your living. These suggestions are going to take complete and thorough effect upon the deepest part of your subconscious mind, sealing themselves in the deepest part of your subconscious mind, so they will remain there forever, and become a permanent part of every cell of your brain and body. You are going to be surprised and amazed just how effective these suggestions are going to be and how much they will become a part of your everyday life, giving you a brand new pattern, brand new thoughts, a brand new method of action, to make you an effective and successful person.

You will make use of a brand new method that you have never used before. You have begun the first positive approach for obtaining a healthy, attractive body, which you desire. You have chosen hypnosis as a positive means to attain this goal, because hypnosis is a great aid in permanently changing your emotional reactions to food and eating. You realize that hypnosis is a new positive approach -- a new positive approach to obtain what you desire.

For the first time in your life you will really initiate a good positive approach toward food and eating. As you initiate this good, positive attitude toward food, enjoy food, like food, eat food. You will create a permanent positive change in your eating habits.

From now on, you will prove to your own satisfaction that eating all you physiologically need will entirely satisfy you; just like drinking all the water you need. Instead of trying to kill your appetite, treating it as an enemy, you are going to work within the framework of your inborn normal reflexes, making a friend of your appetite, paying attention to it; for this is a good thing. Slim people have appetites. They pay attention to them. Attractive people have appetites. They pay attention to them. Hypnosis makes a friend of your appetite, rather than an enemy.

In the past, you've been paying attention only to half the signal from your appetite. Namely, the signal that says, "Eat. I'm hungry." But now you are making a friend of your appetite. You listen to all of what your friend's advice is. When it says "I'm hungry," you eat. When the hunger feeling first disappears, and your appetite says, "I'm satisfied," you stop. You stop long before you're full, because once you have this full sensation; it means that you have grossly overeaten. You should never want to feel full again.

You see you haven't really been paying attention to your appetite at all because your eating has been driven by emotions rather than hunger. It is always proper to eat when your appetite says, "I'm hungry." But you've been eating when you've not been hungry. You've been eating out of habit when your body had no physiological need for food. You've been eating to satisfy psychological, emotional cravings. You haven't paid attention to your appetite when it says "I'm done. I'm satisfied. Stop eating." You haven't paid attention to it either. Your appetite doesn't need killing off. On the contrary, it needs reinforcing. Hypnosis helps you make a friend of your appetite. Pay attention to the advice of your new friend. Tune in on your body sensations. If you eat too much against the advice of your new friend, you'll violate your normal reflexes.

It's important that you should eat all you physiologically need to replace your energy stores for immediate use and to store your body's sugar. You must immediately ban any and all plans that you have for dieting. You will do so. Otherwise, you bring into play an old instinct for self-preservation. This can spoil all of the positive results that you wish to gain from hypnosis. It is important that you develop the habit now; that you're always going to eat all that you need. Under hypnosis, you can reinforce the normal feedback mechanisms, the checks and balances that tell you when you need food and when your appetite is satisfied.

However strong this hypnosis may be, it cannot overcome basic instincts for survival. A most strong instinct is self-preservation. Surprisingly, your great concern about being overweight leads to sporadic dieting. This in turn suggests starvation. Starvation, in turn, demands defense. It brings out the instinct of self-survival. This instinct is responsible for maintaining your excess weight. Slim people eat all they want.

Slim people do well. Slim, attractive people say, "I eat all I want and I don't gain an ounce."

Visualize yourself as this slim, attractive person; the slim, healthy, attractive person that you soon will be. You soon will be saying the very same thing. As you begin to talk and act like a slim, healthy, attractive person, you will soon become one. Overweight is primarily not a dietary problem, but an emotional problem. You must resolve right now to give up dieting forever. You will form a habit pattern to eat all you need when your body needs it. Paying attention to your appetite, trusting your own reflexes, reinforcing the sensation, reflexes and feed-back patterns. This is true even though you may lose very slowly at first. The excess fat will be burned away in due time. You are going to be slim, healthy, and attractive. You will feel wonderful in every way. The word diet and dieting will be removed from your mind and all the plans you may have had for dieting will be removed from your mind thoroughly. Dieting makes you think of growing hungry and giving up food, which in turn starts the anxiety about starvation which brings forth the instinct of self-preservation. So you are through with dieting; through with dieting forever.

Through hypnosis you will restore normal reflexes that will keep you satisfied and bring into play that wonderful feeling of well-being. The word diet is a negative word; it threatens you with denial of food and death. Hypnosis is a positive word; it makes you relax, comfortable and alive. Diets fail; hypnosis succeeds. Diet brings about starvation which leads to overeating and obesity. Hypnosis brings about satisfaction, which leads to relaxation and brings about a slim, healthy, attractive body, a relaxed mind and a satisfied spirit. The old urge to diet is now completely removed from your mind for now you realize that the real answer is in restoring normal reflexes. You will concentrate on it, obeying every suggestion I give you, for hypnosis is a positive approach. Hypnotic suggestions which you receive will rapidly bring about a change which is necessary to insure a permanently slim, healthy, attractive body, which you so desire.

Each time you are tempted to eat or drink anything that you know is wrong for you, you will say "no" and stick by it, because the rewards of becoming slimmer are more important to you than eating the wrong foods.

The rewards of being slender, more desirable, sexier, are more important to you than eating foods that you know are wrong for you.

Weight Reduction II

Weight Reduction Session II

As you go deeper and deeper into relaxation, even deeper and deeper down with every breath you exhale, all the sounds fade away in the distance. You will pay attention only to the sound of my voice, listening carefully to the suggestions that I am about to give you. One thing is very important for you: you are not only going to lose weight, but are permanently going to keep it off. This program is designed so that you will permanently lose all your fat, and become a lean, alert and vigorous person. You will lose all your extra weight and keep it off, easily and comfortably. That means that you are going to be completely reconditioned. You will be a new person, in a new lean form, with new eating habits. Not only will you have these new eating habits, but you will be content and happy with yourself and with these new eating habits. You are going to enjoy life, eating the way nature intended, eating only when you have physiological needs for food and no other time; not only now, but for the rest of your life.

You will:
*Drink lots of refreshing, crisp, clean, cold water all day and before meals.
*Pay attention to your appetite and the feeling of being full which is when you will stop eating.
* This feels good…you feel satisfied…and not stuffed…
*Eat only when you are hungry!!! And ONLY when you are hungry.
*Eat slowly…enjoy the taste…be present…and mindful…
*You will put your fork down while chewing your food. Scoop the next bite only after you have swallowed the food completely.

(You may want to add your own ideas here)

In the past, you were eating more than your body needed for its energy requirements, so that you stored this extra energy as inert fat. Now in order to lose weight and reduce this inert fat, you burn it up as you meet your daily requirements for energy. You eat less than you burn each day. Later, when you are lean, you will eat only that amount that you need for your physiological needs each day. But for right now, you are developing habits to eat less than you're using. We are not giving you a measured diet, for that amount will vary from day to day and depend greatly on your activities. You are going to eat a great deal less than you used to eat in the past, but it will be enough to satisfy you. You will eat less, and you will burn the extra fat. You will turn this inert fat into energy.

Fat by its very nature contains an extremely big amount of stored energy. So, if you burn a little of it each day, you will lose only a little weight each day. Nature designed the fat cells to last a long time so the weight loss must be gradual, but it needs to be consistent. It matters not how long it takes to regain lean proportions, for you will surely get there and permanently stay there, as long as you permanently rearrange your thoughts about eating and your emotions about food. The important thing is that you have changed your habits forever. You emerge as a new person with thoroughly changed ideas, a thoroughly changed image of yourself.

Relax and let all of these suggestions sink into the deepest part of your mind's eye as an image. This image is of good and wonderful food. Food you like. There is plenty of it all around you. There always will be plenty of it. There will always be enough food. There is plenty of food everywhere. With all this food readily available, you will never need to store any more food inside your body. There is plenty of food. There are plenty of the right kinds of food, all the kinds and varieties that your body needs when it needs it. From now on you will eat only the very things your body needs, one day at a time. You are through with storing fat. Fat burdens your heart and organ system. Fat keeps you unhealthy. Fat ruins and shortens your life. There is plenty of food all around you. You never again need to store food in your body that is more than your body needs.

There is in your central brain a small area, which regulates the biochemistry of your body and it controls the amount of fat you store in your body. This control is located in the hypothalamic area of the brain. Your subconscious mind, through the hypothalamus, controls your weight by changing the body's chemistry. Hypnosis can influence your subconscious mind to alter the control of both your appetite and storage of food in the form of fat.

Now while under the influence of hypnosis, I am giving you the suggestion that you will change your body's chemistry so that you can break up the storage of fat and prevent the recurrence of any new and unneeded storages of fat, ugly fat. Fat that has been putting an extra burden and overload on the body. Break up and eliminate forever the unneeded fat stores. Change fat to energy and burn it up. Get rid of it in every way possible. You can see the fat melting away as you use it. The fat is being burned up.

You will now use this stored fat to supply energy. This is extra energy to make you more vigorous. As you are eliminating the excess, you will eat far less each day. You will never need to store fat again. You don't want this fat to ever be replaced. These stores are gone forever. They were burdensome to you. You need to get rid of it. You will only eat small amounts until you full. From this moment on, you are going to eat less, but move more and be more and more active, for you feel better than you have ever felt before. You lose the desire for all but a small amount of food until your weight has come down to a lean size you want. Then you will eat sensibly and correctly the rest of your life.

You have feelings of well-being. You will eat sensibly, get plenty of exercise, and drink plenty of water, which makes you feel healthy, lean, and desirable.

You are losing weight steadily every day. You are slim and shapely. The excess weight is melting off you, just melting away and disappearing. You have a stronger feeling every day that you are in complete control of your eating habits. You picture yourself the way you are going to be soon – slim, lean, shapely and sexy.

Now relax and let all these suggestions take a complete effect upon your -- mind, body, and spirit -- as your subconscious mind corrects your body's chemistry. Let your subconscious mind influence the hypothalamus to make this favorable body change. Let your appetite control center become active and present. Eliminate all that extra harmful fat.

You will:
*Drink lots of refreshing, crisp, clean, cold water all day and before meals.
*Pay attention to your appetite and the feeling of being full which is when you will stop eating.
* This feels good…you feel satisfied…and not stuffed…
*Eat only when you are hungry!!! And ONLY when you are hungry.
*Eat slowly…enjoy the taste…be present…and mindful…
*You will put your fork down while chewing your food. Scoop the next bite only after you have swallowed the food completely.

Weight Reduction III

Weight Reduction Session III

Although sometimes we are quite fearful of change or something new, we are well aware there is no chance for improvement unless there is change. If we have had difficulty in some area, we must change the old patterns. So today, I am suggesting that we do something entirely different from what we usually do. Something that may be quite new to you. Although it is likely that you have done it sometime in the past. Today I am proposing that you let yourself see yourself in perspective. See yourself as others might see you or as you might be seen in history.

When you are away from yourself, even for a few moments, you begin to see yourself in an entirely different light. Temporarily, if you separate yourself in time as well as in physical distance, you can see yourself not only as you are at the moment, but as you were yesterday or even far back in childhood. It is quite possible for you to see yourself proceeding through all the stages of growing to the present time, and even projecting your view of yourself into the future. You are capable of doing this. It is a safe procedure. It is possible because your subconscious mind calculates time and distance differently from the subconscious mind. In the conscious mind, everything is very concrete. The minutes progress in orderly fashion to form hours and days, weeks and years. The subconscious mind works very differently. You live in the present, but if you are suddenly, greatly stressed, you call forth experiences from the past. Your defenses and reactions respond instead to the similar stresses of last year or five years ago.

In other words, in the subconscious mind, your frame of reference is entirely different. You can be in the present, but if something provokes or excites you, in a fraction of a second you can revert to childish or infantile behavior and relive an incident with all the sound, fury and emotion you had the first time you experienced it. In other words, in a fraction of a second you can span the years and relive an incident as vividly as you did the first time.

In exactly the same way, it is possible for you to see some of the future. See yourself as you might be behaving a year or five years from now. Predicting the future is possible because the attitudes you hold about yourself determine your behavior, the friends you choose and situations you create. Even though you may not be able to fill in the names of other people or the precise location, you can predict the kind of situation you will place yourself into because of the attitudes you hold about yourself. Time and place in the subconscious mind is only relative. Your attitude and defenses remain almost unchangeable and they interact with the environment in very much the same way throughout you life.

You can quite easily project yourself temporarily outside of your body as if you were a third person and look back at yourself and your surroundings freed of the usual physical limitations. It is very safe to project yourself in spirit out and beyond your normal physical limitations so you can look back at yourself and understand exactly where you are. This projection is entirely at your under your control. You will find it quite easy to separate much of your spirit and intellect from your body so that you can momentarily be free from your body limitations. From this vantage point, you can see yourself in prospective from birth to present. You will become acutely aware of the program you had to adopt to keep your physical body alive in a world that is so threatening. You will be able to understand the family's interactions with you as you have never before been able to understand.

Best of all, from this detached, safe, vantage point, you can plainly see the defenses that you needed when you were very small. You have now outgrown them just as you have outgrown the need for nursing bottles and diapers.

Projection experience is common to everyone who dreams, for dreams change all the usual limitations of time and space. A good example is awakening abruptly from a very sound sleep and being momentarily confused about where you are. You have had the experience of looking in a three-way mirror in a clothing store and seeing yourself in profile and back view and getting an entirely different perspective of yourself. Another way to get a projection of yourself is to look into a mirror that shows your reflection in another mirror. Then, by changing the angle slightly, you can see one mirror reflecting in another in a whole row of mirrors, almost on to eternity. Now to this picture, you add photographs of yourself in the same pose, but each at a different age of your life. You line them up so that you see yourself in these mirrors at all ages from infancy to the present time. Depending on the angle of the mirrors, you can see yourself projected either into the past or into the future.

Now picture yourself intellectually outside your own body with a clear view of your whole life in perspective. You have in your possession all of the wisdom, all the learning and all the understanding that you have ever gained. In this position, you're now able to influence your own destiny by re-programming and upgrading your attitude and defenses. You let yourself change wherever you see the need for growth and maturity so all your reactions may come up to your expectations as you relinquish your hang-ups.

Hear yourself encouraging your whole being to accept yourself and approve of what you do. Especially see yourself reinforcing the normal eating patterns, to eat only when you are hungry, to see that your appetite is easily satisfied. Picture yourself enjoying food immensely but only in quantities you need to fulfill normal physiological requirements. See yourself overcoming the temptation to eat any extra food. As you observe yourself it becomes easier and easier to pass up unneeded food and drink. Especially note carefully how your need to seek approval from everyone else is disappearing very quickly and progressively. More and more you are approving of what you do.

See yourself also using self-hypnosis as a very powerful and safe force for you. Its effectiveness increases as you let part of yourself be projected beyond your usual body limitations so that you can give yourself suggestions much more effectively as if you were a third person. Again and again you are accepting the suggestion that you eat only when you truly need food and that you are satisfied with basic nutrition. See yourself being increasingly happy with your eating pattern and showing approval of what you do.

Weight Loss

Now take a deep breath ... exhale ... and relax ... just allow everything to let go ... you have no place else to be ... nothing else to do ... but just sit back, relax, and let go completely ... You are here to lose weight and to become healthier ... and the way you are going to lose weight ... beginning right now ... is just by relaxing ... that's right, you are going to sit back ... relax ... and allow yourself to accept all the suggestions ... that I am about to give you ...

If you can accept all the suggestions that are being given to you without being critical of them or without over examining them ... and can follow my instructions exactly as I give them to you, you will lose all the weight you desire and attain your goal weight ... Let me repeat that again so it is perfectly clear ... If you can accept all the suggestions that are being given to you without being critical of them or without over examining them ... and can follow my instructions exactly as I give them to you, you will lose all the weight you desire and attain your goal weight ...

Yes this is a very strong statement to say however in the relaxed state that you are now in, your mind is more open to suggestions than at any other time ... and suggestions given in this state are very effective to the subconscious mind ...

Being in this relax state that you are now in you may be hearing everywhere that I say ... or you may only be hearing bits and pieces. As your mind strays back and forth ... here ... and there ... it doesn't matter whether you're listening to me as I speak or not ... all you need to do is relax ... Your conscious mind may be floating all over with many different thoughts going through it ... however you're subconscious mind hears everything, and always pays attention ... and it is to the subconscious mind that I am speaking to right now ...

From this very moment, starting right now ... You no longer have the urge to overeat or to snack in between meals ... Because healthy, well-balanced meals, more than satisfy your appetite ... and the taste and fragrance of your food are better than ever before ... Rich, heavy, suite, fattening foods and drink just no longer appeal to you ... Because healthy life-giving foods taste wonderful, and fill you up.

From now on you noticeably eat your food slower ... Chewing your food thoroughly ... You put down your fork in between bites and don't pick it up again until the bite in your mouth is gone ... you chew slowly so you can digest your food better and you find that you become full, even though you have eaten much less than before.

Imagine yourself right now, standing in front of you at your goal weight ... Imagine yourself standing there and notice what you are wearing, how you look ... How you feel ... Notice how healthy you are ... Notice the confidence that you have ... Look at yourself, get it clear in your mind, because this is the "goal" you. How much do you weigh in this picture? ... Get that weight clear in your mind ... This is the weight that you feel you can comfortably reach, your goal weight ... See yourself clearly, with as much detail as possible ... This is you, this is your goal ... this is what you will become if you follow all of these instructions, exactly as they are given to you ...

You will find you'll be drinking water more than you ever have before ... water will be there to help you lose weight and to remain healthy. Before every meal, you will drink at least one glass of water ... That wonderful crisp, clear refreshing water will taste great to you ... You'll find yourself craving water more and more each and every day ...

From now on you will eat only healthy meals, not becoming hungry in between meals ... You'll not want to overeat or stuff yourself because you'll feel so much healthier, so much happier, so much more vigorous, without an uncomfortable over filled stomach ... You will eat until you are satisfied, and not until you are stuffed ... You will best accomplished this by eating slowly ... By eating slowly you will not become full as quickly as before ...

When you do snack from now on you will snack on healthy items ... No longer will sweets or unhealthy munchie crunchy foods appeal to you. From now on healthy foods appeal to you and if you find yourself in need of something to eat, you'll search out healthy foods and of course you will drink water.

You'll not lose weight so quickly that it will harm your health, but you will lose weight in a steady constant manner ... and with your new lighter physique you'll find that you have more energy ... Energy that will be needed to be put to good use ... You'll find you can move around more easily and exercise more than you have before ... Everything you do will become easier … and you will want to do more each and every day to increase your health.

No longer do you eat due to boredom ... No longer do you eat just for something to do ... No longer do you eat because you are nervous, tense or frustrated. Negative eating is all part of the past.

From now on, you eat to sustain yourself ... You "eat too live", and not "live to eat", that is all part of the past ... You now get enjoyment from other things rather than just food ... You find that doing healthy fun things, brings you enjoyment ... Eating is just something that you do to get energy so you can continue doing the things you enjoy ...

Each meal that you eat, you'll leave a small portion of food in your plate, that you will then throw away once you are finished ... It is no longer important to eat every morsel of food in your plate ... As you find yourself doing this, more and more you'll find that portion you left in your plate to become more and more ... This will aid you in not eating such large meals ... When you are eating at home you'll leave the food on the stove or the serving area and only bring the food to the table that is in your plate. By not having all the food around you at the table you'll find it easier to eat less. You'll find that by having one plate of food that you will be completely satisfied, even knowing that you have left some food on your plate ... It will give you confidence to know that you can walk away, leaving food on your plate ... confidence that will continue to grow more and more as you proceed toward your goal ...

(Additional personal suggestions can be added here)

You are in control of yourself now and are taking the first step at controlling your eating habits ... right now ... Take control ... Eat healthier ... And attain your goal weight.

IDEAL WEIGHT AND SHAPE

Welcome aboard your enlightening adventure...your time to sit...or lie back more comfortably relaxed for if you once believed you could gratify some of your needs only by eating...excessively...then you can especially enjoy venturing inside you...your wide open frontier of capabilities - you may not yet see - yes -- you can be pleasantly surprised.

When realizing you're in ideal bodily form even though your Life Force inside...only desires to be summoned forth so you're provided the freedom to eat when genuinely hungry... the foods your body really needs...the freedom to eat right...effortlessly... yes - you can enjoy not having to do anything you don't even have to listen to me… because your inner...wiser self is exploring for you your life-transforming adventure.

For you know when you're drifting inwardly... your deeper self can provide transforming dreams – and in those dreams you can venture wherever you desire... to perceive your genuine...slender...nature... even venture deep inside...to the side of the sea... for many find the ocean sea a restoring and renewing force in their lives a place where they feel most alive... and in tune with their true needs... for here you're free to breathe in deeply... the salty scent of the ocean and as you walk cross the moist beach sand... can you hear the lapping of the sea's currents... glistening promisingly...in the sunny beams... glistening with the magical ability to instill you with a new...and more rewarding view of food... and transform you...into the shape you always dreamed... so naturally - since it's such a warm sunny day... why not have fun...wade deeper within... and swim always...in these gently streaming currents... evermore embracing you warmly...securely... for with each rhythmic stroke of your arms... are you swimming more in harmony with the sea pouring warmly right through you... and purifying you of those old...old tendencies - at times you sensed some discomfort – unease ... thoughtlessly...reached for food you really didn't need - presently - these tendencies dissolving...more and more resolved - when dissolving freely...and easily... leaving you free to esteem rightfully your life's high value... your right to lead a more vital .pleasurable life of ease... and free to perceive in those times you used to over...overeat... more rewarding means than food to satisfy...really satisfy your needs... and you are discovering evermore of these...lightly gliding astride this magical sea...deeply supporting your need to live...comfortably free...you might like to swim...toward the shore- for when you emerge from the sea purified...

deeply reborn inside ...how soon before you perceive througl1wiser...more discerning eyes...these new opportunities for you...to realize your desired lean...slender form...and so reassured after your transforming swim...you might like to lie...now lie down...on the soft...sandy shore... naturally savor...your increasing...comfort...for when do you perceive - how the sound as you breathe more slowly...and deeply...more closely resembles the sound of the sea's currents...streaming cadently one...by one upon the shore...how each rise...and fall of your chest and abdomen. Send currents of you own life sea - sweeping warmly through...and soothing you...enlightening your true need to eat...when genuinely hungry those foods your body really needs...surely that once so bloated feeling after those huge meals...perceive your wiser self informing you - you ate too much - imploring you - Hey...I hate to be stuffed...with these heavy foods... truly - must have been a chore laboriously overeating...so presently - as you breathe in deeply - deeply... and now ...let go...in a long...sigh of relief... sense how deeply refreshed...thoroughly gratified you are...to open wide the floodgate of your own life sea... liberate these resurgent currents - your true needs and one of these - when genuinely hungry - you can gratify completely - for in these times...
you need only ride feely astride your gently flowing stream... guiding you to eat slowly...those foods your body really needs... surely now how do you feel - seated before your light, vitalizing meal because instead of soaring fast ahead...and wolfing down your food...as you may have in the past... now you can put everything, on hold...and solely...thoughtfully consider...the value for you here...within this nourishing meal... as you really slow...slow down...now fully chew...and chew each mouthful slowly...and thoroughly... surely - why make haste - when you can now allow your taste buds to savor all the delicious flavor of your nutritious foods... when you can now slow...slow down... and be really gratified...by your satisfying meal. and you may be surprised to find these most nutritious foods quite tantalizing...yes - do you pleasurably discover - even though you might eat less - you enjoy your food now...more than ever before...for as you go...deeply..., sense each '~ding these renewing currents"" sweeping warmly through...and soothing you...guiding you to eat when genuinely hungry...the clean, wholesome foods which nourish your body's tissues - ' guiding you to drink life's own e1ixir...cool glasses of water...as in those childhood days - when you finished play and could run towards water's nearest source... do you feel the same pleasure today when quenching your thirst with plenty of water...whenever you sense your body's real need- eating those nutritious...delicious foods- generously supplying the energy your body needs... for you no longer have to endure past, past times... when you were drugged...sluggish with too much food... that once so bloated sensation... when you ate fattening, greasy, sugary foods... encumbering burdens once weighing you down...for now... in those very times you reached for

food thoughtlessly... you can be deeply renewed... since with each breath – deep – deep how soon before you sense inside... these easing...purifying currents of your own life sea... I your own potent desire to live...actively free... streaming warmly through...and so thoroughly fortifying you can you perceive what your favorite sport...or a activity will be for you're naturally lured outdoors... by your surging desire to flex...and stretch...and move... your need to move freely...with ease... still instilled deeply within your heart... still currently stirring...stirring... incessantly 0 ardently beating – beating till so resurgent – revived -.surely alive - yes - sense your wind...your stamina increasing... your leaner...firmer body moving with so much more ease... likely hard to believe you once over...overate...those too heavy...too greasy...too sugary burdens...for presently - you're genuinely having the time of your life- providing - as freely as you wish - this exquisite activity your body requires... providing your desire to be slender...lean... surely - since you highly value your life - your fight to a more vital .pleasurable life of ease... sense inside...your feeling of swelling pride... as you welcome the triumphant freedom to be reborn... naturally in you deal, physical form... for as you're streaming forward with your own life sea... now how do you feel - asserting your real surging desire... to eat the delicious, nutritious foods which your body requires... when genuinely hungry...when you genuinely have the need... for though there may have been those past...past times... when you sensed some source of unease…thoughtlessly reached to over...overeat... presently - when your body breathes more deeply...deeply... how .soon before past tendencies dissolve freely with your renewing own life sea - streaming warmly forth to soothe you - and guide you...towards more life-giving activities- these new alternatives - far more rewarding... really relieving...any source of unease... really satisfying...deeply satisfying your needs... and isn't it a secure feeling to rely on your potent resource... yes certainly enjoy each opportunity - to be renewed by your own Life Force - pouring forth your one compelling...overwhelming desire to be forever...slender...firm-bodied...lean... and you may have been surprised when finding yourself vitalized in great physical shape... because each engaging day was enjoyed more than ever before... for did you simply feel impatient with fattening meals... because they kept you from partaking in more exciting pursuits... or...did you simply forget to eat any needless wasted food... gratified to discover - you were pleasurably satisfied with the new taste revealed in your nutritious...delicious meals and when you sense this positive expectancy... your Life Force sending you forward... toward a more vital pleasurable life of ease - then each new mom - you're reborn anew to see in your mirror view - the genuine slender you - the person you always knew yourself to be.

WEIGHT LOSS - SPEED UP YOUR METABOLISM

You are feeling very relaxed. In fact, you are aware of your body now, and that your body has mass. You can feel it sinking down deeper into the mattress or chair under its weight... your mind is in complete control of your body, including your muscles. So focus your attention on your feet and toes. There's an energy moving into the soles of your feet, and that energy is relaxing all the muscles in your feet and toes. Feel the muscles relax now.... That energy is moving up into your calves, and as it does, both of your calf muscles become quite loose and relaxed. Feel your calf muscles relax now.... The energy is moving now into your thigh muscles, causing them to simply let go and become loose.

Now let your thigh muscles just hang down off the bone.... now that relaxing energy is moving into your hips and groin, and the muscles there also unwind and become loose and relaxed And now that energy flows into your buttocks, and those muscles also relax.... Feel the energy moving now, and it's moving into your abdominal muscles, waist, and small of your back. As it does, all the muscles there are bathed in relaxing energy, which causes them to unwind like a rubber band letting go...And if your mind is wandering now, that's OK. It just means you're relaxing and feeling very languid. Your unconscious mind is listening very carefully to every word I say. Now that energy is flowing up into your chest and upper back, causing the muscles there to relax and just hang loose.

The energy is moving into your shoulders now, and as the muscles relax, you can feel your shoulders sink down.... And now the energy moves into your arms, hands, and fingers, relaxing all those muscles. You might even feel some tingling in your fingertips as the energy reaches them.... That relaxing energy is now moving into your neck, and if you are holding any tension there, it simply dissipates, allowing the neck muscles to become loose and free.... The energy is now moving into your head, causing the muscles on your scalp and around your ears to unwind and it may even feel like your scalp is sliding down.... Now the energy is flowing around your face, and as it moves, all the tiny muscles around your eyes, nose, and mouth let go. Your jaw relaxes and your teeth are slightly parted... Your entire body is now totally relaxed, and your body feels as limp as a rag doll. You are feeling drowsy, and comfortable, and secure. That energy is still in you and is now flowing out the top of your head and is moving down towards your feet. As it reaches your feet, your entire body is now enveloped in a warm cocoon of energy that protects you from any negative influences.

You are very relaxed now, and feeling sleepy.... You may hear sounds in your environment, but unless there's something that needs your immediate attention, you remain totally relaxed. In fact, the sounds you hear, including my voice, only serve to help you go deeper asleep. You have the ability to come out of this trance whenever you wish, and you are fully safe and secure. So continue to fully relax, let go, and be at ease.... You are drifting deeper asleep with every breath you exhale deeper asleep... ever deeper asleep.

Deep inside your mind is the blueprint for a slimmer, healthier you.

Just as your mind had the capacity to add weight to your body, it also has the equal capacity to reduce your body weight—effectively, easily—and your mind does this by accepting these wonderful new ideas about losing weight.

And when your mind accepts these new ideas to reduce weight, your mind normalizes your metabolism, and your daily choices and habits begin to automatically move towards a slimmer, healthier you. These new choices then become easier and easier to become habits - such as eating well, exercising regularly, and releasing unhealthy habits from your life.

Your powerful subconscious mind contains the inner blueprint, which is like the software for your body's computer. This 'programming' for your metabolism and the 'automatic software' creates your everyday habits, which greatly influence body weight - this is the source where new thoughts and ideas originate from, which in turn begin to make changes to your metabolism and your weight.

Your first meal of the day starts your metabolism. Your metabolism then speeds up for 8 hours before gradually slowing down—until its time for you to go to sleep. Whenever you skip breakfast your metabolism doesn't get started until lunchtime, therefore you lose 3 hours of fat burning time. So, in order to lose weight quickly you begin to eat small, regular meals. Whenever you are hungry, you eat a small amount of healthy, nutritious food—and when you've had enough to eat, you stop eating.

You begin to drink more water. Each and every day you're drinking more and more lovely clean, fresh, cold water. Water becomes the only drink that truly satisfies your thirst, it becomes a drink you really do enjoy, and you begin a new healthy habit of drinking a glass of cool refreshing water before each meal. This glass of cool clean fresh water slightly shrinks your stomach, so that you find yourself eating less, yet feeling fuller. You're eating less, yet feeling fuller. You also begin walking more.

You begin to use your body, and the more you use your body, the healthier and slimmer you become. From now on you much prefer walking than driving a car, and if you can walk, instead of taking the car, or any other form of transport, then you much prefer to do so.

You love the feeling of tightness in your muscles after a nice brisk walk; this reminds you that you're losing weight. You're losing weight and feeling great— you're losing weight and feeling wonderful. You're becoming slimmer and healthier and fitter, each and every day.

And every day you use your self hypnosis in order to speed up your metabolism. And I want you to imagine now that you are a work person, with a torch in one hand and a bag of tools in the other, and that you're going up into your powerhouse subconscious mind. Use your imagination and visualize the scene I describe to the very best of your ability. Make it real, perceive any sounds or smells that may come into your awareness. And imagine a long staircase leading up into the control room—the staircase has 20 steps leading up, and you begin to walk up the steps, into the control room. I'm going to count the steps up and you will find yourself going up, and up and up. Up into the control room where your metabolism, amongst other things, is regulated.

So, when you are ready, begin to walk up the staircase, counting with me as we go up.

1 -- 20.

Now you're entering a large and comfortable room. In the room are many panels which have switches and levers, they have buttons and knobs. They are various shapes and sizes. Take a look around. Nod when you can see them.

Good. Now look for a label which says 'metabolism'' Make your way over to it and take a really good look at the switch or knob or lever or button or whatever you see.

Now your task is easy. We know that for some reason your metabolism has slowed down to how it used to be. The switch or knob or lever or button must be stuck somehow, or perhaps it's broken or maybe needs oiling or adjusting in some way. You have a bag of tools and you can do, whatever you need to do, to adjust your metabolism, to make it work, how it used to work.

So using the language of the brain, your wonderful imagination, I want you to make the necessary adjustments to your metabolism, to speed it up, to make it work more effectively, so that it burns up the excess fat that is stored in your cells.

I know that you can do this, in your own, wonderful way. So I'm going to be quiet for a few moments to allow your mind to work in a way that it knows is best for you.

PAUSE.

Have you finished? Good. Now take a look at your work, test it, and see how you have adjusted it to the correct setting, to enable fat to be burned more quickly and easily. Now on one side of the room is a lovely, full length mirror. Take a walk over to the mirror and see a reflection of yourself as you are now. Examine your body from head to toe, the front, the back the sides. Now you have a good strong, healthy body, a wonderful body, and you like your body and you love your body. You love and respect your body, and all you need to do is to lose some of that excess weight that you've been carrying around for so long. And even as you continue to gaze at your reflection in the mirror, I want you to see the fat beginning to melt away. To disappear, until, your body moves into the proportion and dimension that you desire, Your perfect self.

I'm going to count from one to five. At the count of five you'll be wide awake.

One, two, three, four, five.

HYPNOTIC STOMACH STAPLING

You are now deeply relaxed and the suggestions that you hear will have a permanent and immediate effect on your subconscious mind - you will hear every word that I speak - even though you may find your mind wandering away at times - because right now - nothing else matters - nothing - except for this wonderful feeling of relaxation that you're experiencing.

At this moment is as though you haven't a care in the world - nobody wants anything - nobody needs anything - there is absolutely nothing at all for you to do except relax and let go - and just enjoy the feelings that are being generated within you.

Because - for a while now you've been feeling fed up with all the excess weight that you've been carrying around. So much so that you've been thinking about taking drastic measures to loose that weight and keep it off – you've even considered stomach stapling!

But did you know that with the power of your subconscious mind – you can do anything - your mind can control almost every aspect of your body. From simple things such as walking and holding your breath, to more complex issues such as blushing or hay fever. All you have to do is believe in the power of your own subconscious mind.

So today we will perform a stomach stapling operation, but using only the power of your subconscious mind – for your subconscious mind is more powerful than you can ever imagine. And the result of this operation is that you will start to eat less – as you would naturally expect after this operation, and so the weight will start to drop of you. The benefit of this hypnotic stomach stapling is that you will not experience any of the side effects from the real operation, you will not have to recover from the surgery – and the results will be instantaneous!

So I want to imagine that you are a very, very small person. You are so light that you can float in the air – the slightest breeze blows you one way or the other. As you are floating around, you are looking down on yourself, seeing your relaxed body. You are drifting closer and closer, until you can feel the air going in and out of your lungs. Suddenly, with one strong breath, you get sucked into your nose. There is nothing you can do to stop yourself – you have no control over your physical body and there is nothing for your tiny body to grab hold of. It is as if you are on a roller coaster, you are getting sucked closer and closer to your body, you can smell your aroma, as you get close to your body – and then all of a sudden – pop you have entered your own body.

You get sucked in through your nose. It is very dark and you can't see anything, but the hairs in your nose tickle you as you go past them. You try to grab hold of them, but they are too wet and slippery and you are going too fast – there is nothing you can do but to relax and let yourself go.

You get through your nasal cavity and suddenly the wind stops and you are diverted down your food pipe and into your stomach. Your eyes have still not adjusted but you can feel yourself going down and down.

Eventually, you come to an abrupt stop – you have landed of a soft, damp spongy surface – it is very bouncy and you go up and down a couple of time before coming to a rest.

The smell of your stomach is acidic and slightly unpleasant, but you soon get used to it ad before you know it, you have forgotten about the smell completely. Your eyes start to adjust to the darkness and now you can see clearly around you.

Except there isn't much to look at. You are in quite a large cave –your stomach. The walls are saggy – like bits of material that haven't been secured properly and there are a few remains of your last meal on the floor. You are glad that it has been a while since you last ate, else you would be wading through food.

Now you have come down here to fix a problem – your excessive eating – and that is exactly what you will do.

You have come equipped with a hand stapler – a bit like the kind they use at school to pin up posters on the walls.

You walk over to the wall, and lift up one of the folds of skin to examine it. You see immediately how it works. When you eat a big meal, your stomach expands to fit it all in, and these flaps of skin get stretched out to their full potential. You know that you do not need your stomach to become this big, it only encourages you to eat more to fill it up, and so putting on weight.

So you start to work stapling these flaps of skin to the walls of your stomach. Then next time you have a meal, your stomach will be unable to expand, and so you will have to stop eating sooner – when you run out of room in your stomach.

You staple the first flap up – it takes a few staples, but finally it is up and secure. You set about, stapling all the other flaps to the sides of your stomach wall, and the more you do the faster and more efficient you become at it.

Before you know it, all the flaps have been stapled up, and the inside of our stomach looks a bit like a patchwork quilt cover. But this is OK, because given a bit of time; these flaps will slowly melt into the sides of your stomach wall and become part of them. If you were to come back here in a year's time, you would never know that your stomach had ever been so big.

You look around you and admire your work – you've done a pretty good job, even if you say so yourself.

Now it's time to make your way out of your stomach and in to the outer world. This time it's much easier than before, you stand underneath the food pipe and simply take a big jump up, there is enough bounce in your stomach to take you all the way up. You bounce up, up and away, up through your food pipe and your nostril to the big outside world. The light is dazzling, but you soon get used to it and then you can see your relaxed self below you. You gently float down and rejoin with your physical self.

The memory of how flabby your stomach was stays with you and is a permanent reminder never to eat excessively again.

The trip into your stomach also motivates you to start to make the most of life and look after your body really well. You eat so much healthier. By eating well, you can enjoy a higher energy level and ability to exercise, and thus a healthier weight. You make the most of every mouthful that you do eat – making sure that it is full of goodness and nutrients and try your best to avoid bad foods. You take plenty of time to eat, eating slowly and chewing each mouthful well, and you respond immediately when your stomach sends the signals to your brain to say that it is full.

You start to enjoy taking brisk energetic walks in the park or wood. You increase your energy levels in every way possible, for although your stomach is now fixed, you still have excess weight to loose and this will take time. But by taking small amounts of exercise, you will find the excess weight soon drops off and thanks to your smaller stomach, it stays off. You are in overall better shape and this sets you going in an upward circle, feeling better and better all the time.

Before you know it, you will have reached your ideal weight and most of all; you will have complete control over the amount of food that you eat.

And every day you find that you feel better and happier and healthier.

And these suggestions are firmly embedded in your subconscious mind and grow stronger and stronger day by day.

In a moment I'm going to count from one to five and at the count of five you'll be wide, wide-awake.

One, two, three, four, five.

HEALTHY EATING

For a long time now you've been filling your body with junk food - missing out on the important vitamins, minerals and roughage that your body requires - but now - you've decided to do something about it - that's why you're here.

You're beginning to realize more and more - that there's a better way - a healthier way of living. Like anything in life - you only get out - what you put in. Just think about it - if you put inferior fuel into a brand new car it wouldn't perform too well - it would stall and be sluggish and wouldn't accelerate to its peak performance - leading to all sorts of problems with the car.

Similarly - when you're baking an extra special dish you want only the finest ingredients to give just the right taste.

I know you've been put off by the taste and texture of healthy foods in the past - but all that is changing now - not overnight - you won't suddenly wake up one day and eat lots and lots of fruit and vegetables and salads - that would be foolish to change so rapidly - your digestive system wouldn't understand what was happening to it. No - you're going to change your eating habits gradually and easily - trying one new thing at a time.

And more and more you'll find yourself rejecting the old, inferior junk food that you used to eat - in favor of a healthier selection - not by magic or miracles - not because I say so - but because you have already decided you want this change - your body has been crying out for healthier foods - and it's finally got through to your mind to do something about it.

But first I want you to go back in time - to your earliest years - and remember a time in those past - faraway childhood days - when you were filled with a sense of curiosity. As infants that's how we found out about things in the world - first we become curious and were driven by an overwhelming desire to discover for ourselves - what we needed to experience.

I once knew a small child who felt just like that - there was a sideboard in the best room of her house - the room which children weren't allowed into very often - and in that sideboard was a set of drawers - and the top drawer contained all manner of memorabilia . She was only a small child and whenever she got the chance she would carry a stool and climb up and spend hours rooting through that drawer.

And each little button or photograph she found had its own little story to tell - her imagination would create stories about what she'd discovered - she was just driven by curiosity - that's how children are.

And I wonder if you can remember that time when you felt something like that - recapture that feeling now - hold it there in your heart and take a deep breath - whilst your subconscious mind memorizes that feeling - and bring it back with you to your present age.

In the future when you see different foods - fresh foods - a myriad of colored vegetables, crisp and clean, tossed green and mixed salads sprinkled with herbs and marinated in wine vinegar or lemon juice and freshly ground black pepper and exotic fruit - like mangos and kiwi and papayas- you'll find that this same sense of curiosity will overtake you - you will become fascinated by the thought of how they taste - and the only way to satisfy that curiosity will be to actually taste that good food.

Each time you may find something different to taste - perhaps one day you'll want to eat an juicy fresh orange - another day you may wonder how green broccoli tastes - or all those other good foods that you previously wouldn't eat. And once the thought comes into your mind - you'll feel a strong desire to discover for yourself - how delicious that natural healthy food is.

And you'll soon find yourself eating many varieties of succulent fruit and vegetables and salad - and you can become curious about how long it will take before you totally reject that old way of life - in favor of healthy living. There is an infinite menu of combinations which only you can experiment with. And very soon you'll discover which your favorites are - and you'll be eating them more and more.

In a moment I'm going to count from one to five and at the count of five you'll be wide awake, you'll have beautiful feelings flowing through your body, calm and peaceful thoughts flowing through your mind.

One, two, three, four, five.

WEIGHT LOSS - CONTROL ROOM

Visual imagery is the language of the brain – and you're going to use your wonderful rich imagination now – and visit the control room of your mind. You imagine walking into the control room and suddenly you're surrounded by panels with switches and buttons and knobs and colored lights of different shapes and sizes.

There is a higher control room which can be reached by climbing five steps and the door is closed.

You climb the steps to the higher control room and push open the door. Now you are in a room similar to the one below, but here it's more like a laboratory with rows and rows of taps and tubes, all carefully labeled and put into alphabetical order. The switches are labeled too, and you look around until you find the letter 'M' and a round knob, which is attached to a drawer that is labeled – metabolism.

You notice that the knob has worked loose and so you gently pull out the drawer. Inside the drawer are phials containing hormones and one of them is nearly empty. Like a scientist you take it to the tubes or taps and carefully fill it up with the correct hormone. Somehow you seem to know exactly which hormone you need. Then you carefully replace the phial back into the drawer and close it, tightening the knob as you do so.

And as you do this, an amazing thing begins to happen. The chemicals in your brain become regulated and you feel a warm inner glow deep within you. You can really notice it now. You can feel and experience that warm inner glow – tiny at first but then spreading within your body. Because you're going to find that you have more energy, more vitality, you feel younger and fitter and healthier, and every day this feeling within you grows stronger.

Returning to the dials and switches in the control room you notice that one of the dials is labeled 'Appetite' and that this dial is set much higher than it needs to be. Carefully you ease the dial backwards in an anticlockwise movement because you are aware that there is always plenty of food, and you don't need or want to eat as much as you used to do. And as your hand moves the dial in this backward movement a surprising thing happens to you. You feel deep within you, a contentment, a feeling of satisfaction in your stomach as you realize that you only need to eat small amounts of food to satisfy your needs.

And good feelings spread throughout your body, and your mind, because you're eating less now, but deriving the same sense of satisfaction as when you used to eat more. And it's good to eat less than you need, your stomach begins to enjoy a lighter feeling as it flattens and shrinks and your waist becomes trimmer and neater, which gives you a feeling of confidence in yourself. Because you realize now that you're in control of yourself. When you have had enough to eat you stop eating, and it's so easy to stop eating and enjoy a lighter feeling of satisfaction within you.

And again, as you look around the control room you notice that there are switches connected to Taste. Some of these switches are set in the wrong position. For example there may be a switch regulating your taste for sweet foods or drinks, and if this is set up too high you find that you can adjust it, and in doing so you adjust your own natural taste and desire as you begin to enjoy healthier foods and drinks. The switches may indicate that in the past you have eaten too much fat and need to reduce this for the benefit of your health and your body. The mere thought of fat fills you with disgust as you imagine fatty greasy layers floating up through your body to the surface of your beautiful skin, clogging up the pores of your skin, which needs to breathe as it is a living organ on your body.

You adjust the switch in a way that your subconscious mind automatically knows is correct for you. And in doing so you soon begin to notice that fatty, greasy foods taste ten times fattier and greasier than they ever did before. Therefore your mind and your body reject all fatty, greasy foods.

You may discover that there are healthy foods that you have avoided in the past, perhaps certain fruits or salads or fresh, crisp vegetables. Maybe the switches need regulating to help you to regain your natural taste buds and enjoy these wonderful, healthy foods. And you find that everything you put into your mouth, turns into health and beauty. Everything that you eat, from this forward, is good for you, otherwise you wouldn't eat it. You enjoy eating small amounts of healthy food, for that satisfies you completely, and that satisfies you completely.

You may see a mirror in your control room with a distorted image of yourself. And as you move toward the mirror you begin to see your reflection and discover that this image can change and become you as you really want to be. Slim, healthy, attractive, looking serene and calm, relaxed and happy. You may even notice the clothes that you are wearing and how good they look on your slimmer, wonderful body. This makes you feel good.

Another switch may represent the word Energy and it's possible that in the past your energy levels were low because of the excess weight that you were carrying. But now you realize that you're on your way to becoming the person that you desire to be and this motivates you to exercise and move around in a way that actually creates a more positive energy in you.

And in the past, if you were one of those people who used to drive everywhere they went, you may now even find a great pleasure in walking whenever you can. You enjoy movement, moving your body in a graceful way and knowing that you're looking better and healthier every single day. You may find other forms of exercise that are beneficial to you, and discovering new ways of using your body becomes a source of inspiration to you. Your exercises are always gentle and you allow your body to warm up first, proceeding in a manner that is safe and comfortable for you.

There may be a switch that represents the word Comfort - and if you've ever found that eating comforts you in some strange way - then you can turn off that switch now as you realize that it was a false comfort and in fact - only led to heavy, uncomfortable feelings in your stomach. You can feel more satisfied on smaller amounts of food and more comfort by asking yourself what you really need - and if it's company you seek a more realistic way of satisfying this need. If it's love then you also realize that overeating and gaining weight is counter productive to your desire for to gain love - you must first love yourself. And you are learning to do this right now in hypnosis, as you go deeper into relaxation.

And as you become your own person, slimmer and healthier and happier of course, you realize that you are also becoming a much more confident person.

This is not simply because of the weight that is coming off you, but because you realize now that you are in control. You have a healthy and active mind and you are careful about the sort of thoughts that your mind thinks. You do not allow yourself, or anyone else, to put you down, because you realize that you are a very special person, a wonderful human being, and if any negative thoughts do enter your mind, your are instantly on vigil, and push the thoughts out of your mind, replacing them with more positive thoughts.

Because of all this you find that you are smiling more. You feel happier, more relaxed, more comfortable with yourself as the wonderful individual that you are. Your happier thoughts produce good feelings within you and these good feelings become stronger and stronger as each wonderful day goes by.

You're becoming a slimmer and healthier and happier person – a much more confident person – and those around you are astonished in the changes to your personality because you inject enthusiasm and love and motivation to those that you meet. You feel good about yourself and you feel good about other people. This means that other people feel good about themselves and they also feel good about you.

And these wonderful, positive changes are beginning to take place now at a deeper level of mind. They will continue to take effect and grow stronger and stronger as each moment goes by.

Now I'll count to five and at the count of five I want you to come all the way back.

One, two, three, four, five.

Eyes open, wide awake.

WEIGHT LOSS (NLP TYPE APPROACH)

Go ahead now and take a deep breath. And just allow that breath to exhale slowly and focus your attention now on someone whom you know has skills, abilities, and resources that you'd like to have -especially the skills, the resources, and the abilities to say "No" to food between meals.

And when you've thought of this person, I want you to imagine that person at a distance as though you're watching them from a distance, move through the amount of their day.

And when you have them in your mind, just let your right index finger lift gently up so that I know, (pause for response) good.

Imagine, from a distance, that you're watching them move through the amount of their day. They're moving through activities and encounters...people are offering them food...and, perhaps, offering inappropriate drinks, and they're simply saying "No, thanks."

It's just natural, it's normal, and it's expected by them. Others expect them to act and treat them that way, - even though they're offering — because that's what they do—it's the right thing for them to do, to offer. And it is the right thing for you to do to say "No."

As you move through the experience, notice one of the days when they've eaten the right foods at the right time and in the right sequence. And most importantly, I want you to notice, from a distance, how they stop eating when they're full...how natural it is for them to leave food on their plate. And when you've watched them through the amount of their day—mentally taking all the time that you need, just like you're watching a movie, perhaps, about someone who has the behaviors and attitudes and beliefs that you're acquiring now—just give me a "yes" response...(pause for response)...that's right.

Now, imagine that you could step back and start that day over again, but this time imagine the possibility of stepping into their body. Imagine what it might be like if you could see through their eyes, hear with their ears, and sense and feel with their body, and understand, by walking in their shoes, how it is they do what they do. Imagine, just for a moment, that you could listen to their internal dialogue...that you could hear them communicate with themselves about food...about what people are saying...and most importantly, listen to their positive, dynamic internal dialogue. Notice how natural it is for them to look down at their body and honor and love and appreciate their body.

And when you've moved through that same day now, differently, by seeing through their eyes, hearing through their ears, and sensing and feeling what their body is sensing and feeling so that you can acquire those skills in a new way, just give me a "yes" response so that I know...that's right.

Now, imagine, that you could bring all of those skills and abilities back into your body right here and right now...that those skills, those abilities, and those resources could stretch out into your body right here...that you could feel them surging from your heartbeat all the way down to the bottom of the feet...that you could feel them moving to the tips of your fingers...that you could feel them integrating through the legs and the arms. You could feel them in their own unique way integrating into your lifestyle. And imagine, (client's name), three places where you'd want to benefit from those new behaviors, attitudes, and beliefs in the next week...and you've lost from one to three pounds a week, and it was easy and natural for you, just give me a "yes" response so that I know...(pause)...that's right.

And now, as you think of that week again, think of ways you can make the next week even more fun and easy. Imagine, like a producer, you could place greater joy, greater happiness, and greater harmony by placing your favorite music in the background...as if someone has taken your life and made a script for health, harmony, and vitality. And when you've made it through the day in this way, just give me a "yes" response so that I know...that's right.

Step into the future. Imagine that you're there a week from today and you've done it...one more week and you've lost one to three pounds. Notice the joy that your body is experiencing by losing one pound a week, knowing that you will never ever have to lose that pound again...that it's permanent, natural, and forever. That pound no longer serves or produces results for you, so you converted the energy into a dynamic, positive attitude...for all energy changes shape and form, and now, in your mind, it's changing to a shape and a form which is more productive, more positive, and more permanent for you...a permanent, lasting change where your shoulders will roll back, your chin will roll upward, and you will feel extremely good for no apparent reason. The days themselves will transform into weeks and the weeks into months and the months into years.

It is from here that as you concentrate your attention on my voice that all outside sounds, all outside influences will simply dissolve, dissipate, and melt away. It is from here that I want you to imagine your favorite vacation, and just take a mental trip where you can take care of all the stress, strain, and confusion once and for all and permanently for today. Just let the stress go by taking a mental vacation where the seconds become hours. And when you've taken all the time that you need on that mental vacation so that, upon awakening today, you can be rested, relaxed, revitalized, and renewed...ready to treat people with more love, with more respect, with more integrity than you ever have before...just give me a "yes" response so that I know...that's right.

Now, with that mental attitude in mind, as you journey deep, deep inside, is there any part of you at all that objects in you utilizing this process known as the unlimited reality where you can learn from others vicariously, the same way you learned as a child, but this time you get to pick and choose your teachers by choosing people in the world around you that have skills and benefits and behaviors that you truly want, but you could use them and benefit from them through a process of osmosis where it would simply happen for you without question or hesitation upon awakening. Is there any part of you at all that would object in you acquiring positive, beneficial behaviors for every area of your life so improvements can be made everywhere?

Excellent. Just know, if there was a part of you that would object to this process, that that part of you would be taken deep, deep inside...deep, in fact, to the very core of your mind where it would be explained about the new behaviors, the new attitudes, and the new beliefs and how a synergizing effect is happening in your mind...synergizing, meaning that every part is necessary and needed, that as your body as a perfectly-tuned organism works together, you will take the weight off and keep it off forever.

It is from here, (client's name), that I want you to look forward to the future. Given the information that you're learning here, one day at a time, and the continuing training that you will be receiving, do you feel that you're getting the information you need to take the weight off and keep it off forever? (Pause)

Just know that if for any reason your unconscious or conscious mind feels that you're not getting what you need, all you would need to do is say so in the state of hypnosis, and then the appropriate behavior, the appropriate attitude, the appropriate learned experience would be given to you without question, without hesitation so that every day, in every way, greater joy, greater happiness, and greater harmony can start first in your mind and then flow freely through your thoughts and then become a part of your everyday reality. The days transforming into weeks, the weeks transforming into months, and the months transforming into years. It is from here, (client's name), that the days become weeks and the weeks become months and the months become years.

So that you can receive the benefits that you want today, and they will only improve upon awakening, I say to you now, focus on your breathing. If this is a time of sleep for you, (client's name) , then you will continue the journey into deep, restful, relaxing sleep where you dream of all of the people that you've ever seen, heard, or had experiences with that had skills, behaviors, or attitudes that you would like to acquire. And because you've done the process once here, you can continue to do the process deep, deep inside in your dreams so that, upon awakening, spontaneous, natural changes can take place...positive changes. I say to you now, negative thoughts, negative influences, negative beliefs will have no control over you at this or any of the awakening levels of consciousness. You will only accept and use that which is positive, productive, life-giving and forgiving for you.

So the benefits will be multiplied upon awakening, I say to you now, if this is a time and a place where you need to be awake, alert, and conscious, then you will slowly find yourself returning back into the room...slowly finding yourself returning back into the room where your eyes will open, you will become wide awake...feeling fine and in perfect health...feeling better than ever before, perhaps feeling as if you've just returned from a deep, relaxing, powerful mental holiday.

WEIGHT LOSS MAINTENANCE

You are now deeply relaxed and the suggestions that you hear will have a permanent and immediate effect on your subconscious mind - you will hear every word that I speak - even though you may find your mind wandering away at times - because right now - nothing else matters - nothing - except for this wonderful feeling of relaxation that you're experiencing.

At this moment is as though you haven't a care in the world - nobody wants anything - nobody needs anything - there is absolutely nothing at all for you to do except relax and let go - and just enjoy the feelings that are being generated within you.

Congratulations!! You've lost the weight you've been working so hard to lose. Now, you want to keep it off.
And you CAN keep it off – you've done the really hard part of losing the weight in the first place – now you want to cling onto that new slim figure of yours.

The power to stay slim lies within yourself – it is within your grasp, and to start with, a few simple life changes, which I'm sure you had to make to lose the weight, in the first place, will help enormously. And by reminding your subconscious mind of these changes, you will find them happening easily and effortlessly

The first thing to do is to keep an eye on your weight. Either use a tape measure to keep tabs on your weight or weigh yourself either once or twice a week. In order to maintain your weight you need to know how much you weigh.

And if you do gain one pound or two, make the changes today that will aid you in taking off that one pound or two. You know how to lose weight, you've done it before. And you know that it will be easier to lose it now than in a few months or years time.
You continue to make exercise part of your everyday routine. Regular exercise means that you will maintain that weight loss. And you did find that whilst losing

your initial weight, you actually enjoyed the exercise – your heart beating faster, pumping more blood around your body, burning up more calories.

In fact it was so good, that I want you to imagine the motions of that exercise right now. Whether it be going for a jog, using the machines at the gym, or even cleaning your floors.

Imagine your muscles moving in exactly the same way they would if you were doing that exercise. Imagine your heart beat increasing slightly and your breathing becoming heavier – all this means that you are working hard, and that you are achieving your ultimate gain – a beautiful slim figure.

You can imagine that your stomach is like a furnace, whenever you exercise, more and more fat is thrown into the fire, all the fat from the places you didn't want it in your body – gone forever.

And now that you have actually lost that weight – this furnace is helping to prevent a build up of fat like before. Helping to keep you slim – exactly the way you are.

Can you remember how you used to look? Can you remember how much you used to wish that you were slim?

Your desire to be slim was so strong that sometimes it hurt. Gradually you lost your weight, and gradually you forgot how much you had wanted to lose weight – because your mind has the ability to forget painful experiences to protect yourself. However in this case, that memory is one that you want to hang onto – to keep at the front of your mind – for the motivation you felt that helped you to lose the weight in the first time will also help you to keep the weight off – forever.

Memories are like balloons, if you don't hold onto them tight, they can drift away. And since you need that memory of how you used to be, and how you used to feel, I want you to find the balloon that represents it and hold on tight to it – perhaps even tying the piece of string that it is attached to part of your body – for you know that it is there to help you.

And if ever you lapse into bad habits, all you have to do is remember how much you wanted to lose the weight in the first place – and how much you want to keep it off – forever.

You continue to eat regular healthy meals, always watching your portion sizes and never over indulge, although a small treat occasionally is also ok if you choose, since you worked so hard – perhaps you can do an extra half hour of exercise to compensate.

You know what suits your body the best, you learnt so much during the time you were losing your weight, and so you can tailor your lifestyle to these needs.

You now lead a healthy lifestyle and are so glad that you made these changes when you did and stuck to them, for now your future also looks healthy. You can enjoy your older years and be healthy and active, instead of sitting in a rocking chair, talking about your ill health.

The rest of your future looks rosy, you know that it will be healthy; for you are determined to keep off that weight, and do everything you can to help yourself. Because you look so good now that you lost the weight and you are going to stay the same - forever

And these suggestions are firmly embedded in your subconscious mind and grow stronger and stronger each and every day. You become a much healthier person, and love the body you are in. If you feel unmotivated then all you need do is to remember how you used to be – and how desperate you were to lose that weight – and then how happy you are to know that you reached your goal.

And in a moment I'm going to count up from one to five and at the count of five you'll be wide awake, but these suggestions will grow stronger by the day, stronger by the hour, stronger by the minute.

So get ready now as I count up to five and come all the way back at the count of five.

One, two, three, four, five.

CHOOSING THE RIGHT THERAPIST

Choosing the right therapist is a crucial first step. I encourage you to ask many questions and if the therapist seems offended, question it! Choose a professional who you feel comfortable with and who will support your goals. If you practice a specific religion, you may want to work with a therapist who can support you in your faith. Choose a therapist who speaks your preferred language. Make sure the therapist has experience helping couples work through relational and marital issues. It is also important to know that the therapist completed a supervised clinical experience and is governed by a licensing board or other credentialing organization. Some common designations include: MA, MS, MSW, LMHC, MFT, NCC, PhD, PsyD. The type of credential may not be as important as some may believe. For example, a LMHC may be just as good a therapist as a PsyD or PhD.

If you do not have a referral for a therapist you may want to start by calling a few and conducting a brief interview to find out key information about services offered and expertise. Unless the therapist has time to speak, do not expect the first phone consultation to be too extensive. You may have the opportunity to give your name, referral source, phone number, and to ask a few basic questions. If you do not feel comfortable setting up an appointment ask the therapist to call you back when she has more time to answer more questions. A question to help ease anxiety about going to your first therapy session is simply to ask what to expect in your first meeting so that you are able to prepare yourself.

During the initial session with a therapist, pay attention to your comfort levels and the feel of the setting where you will be engaging in therapy. Be sure that the therapist can accommodate certain times that you have available to meet. It may also be beneficial to know what the therapist's policy is regarding appointment cancellations and make-up sessions. Also, you may want to find out what the therapist's accessibility between sessions and phone contact policy entails. Ask about the fee, method of payment preferred, and if there is a sliding scale. Many mental health professionals offer 'sliding-scale' fees – or prices based on your income or ability to pay. Pay attention to whether or not you feel that you and the therapist are a good match. Be sure that you felt heard and that you can be open and trust the therapist. It is worth your money and time to find the most suitable therapist for you and your partner. Research on successful outcomes in therapy has found one consistent finding time and time again: individuals feel that therapy was successful based on the quality of the relationship with their therapist. If the therapist is able to build a trusting, healthy relationship with you, he or she should be able to help the you achieve your desired goals.

Unlike medicine and medical doctors, where the curative medicine is independent of the provider, the personality of the psychotherapist plays a significant role in the healing work. In other words, not all therapists are the same nor do they approach your concerns in even remotely the same way and this difference matters. It is very important for you to feel you have the right fit with the person whom is going to accompany you on your healing journey. An extra word of caution is important here. Don't expect yourself to immediately feel comfortable with any therapist, if this is your first time in therapy. Starting therapy can be anxiety producing for you and it would be a mistake to prematurely judge the fit. You and your potential therapist might agree to meet for a couple of sessions to see if things settle down and the comfort increases.

These are the characteristics I'm looking for in a therapist:

1.

2.

3.

4.

5.

I'd be willing to compromise on:

1.

2.

3.

But I won't compromise on:

1.

2.

3.

QUESTIONS FOR A POTENTIAL THERAPIST

Once you've come up with your list of wants, turn that list into questions:

1.

2.

3.

4.

5.

6.

7.

8.

9.

10.

Referrals

If you would like a referral to a specially trained professional who may be able to help you overcome the issues discussed, please call my office for assistance:

Dr. Elizabeth Mahaney (813) 240-3237

elizabethmahaney@msn.com

www.SouthTampaTherapy.com

425 S. Orleans Ave.

Tampa, Fl 33606

Or call The Missing Piece of Counseling & Well-Being, Inc.- A non-profit organization.

(813) 240-3237

www.MissingPieceCounseling.org

425 S. Orleans Ave.

Tampa, FL 33606

TERMS OF SERVICE AND USE

TERMS OS SERVICE FOR YOUR OWN PERSONAL USE

Welcome, by using our web site, products or services you agree to be bound by the following terms and conditions (the "terms of Service or Use").

PERSONAL USE ONLY

Our web site, products or services are made available for your personal, non-commercial use only. You may not use our web site, products or services to sell a product or service, or to increase traffic to your web site for commercial reasons, such as advertising sales. You may not "meta-search" our web site, products or services. If you want to make commercial use of our products or services, you must enter into an agreement with us to do so in advance. Please contact us for more information.

MEDIA

You may copy and use segments of up to 150 words of text from our web site, products or services for reviews or for non-profit educational purposes but such use must be accompanied by the following acknowledgement on the same document so that everyone knows from where it came, and none of my text be

modified or altered in any way.

From *Lose Weight Now! A Manual For Weightloss*, © copyright 2009, by Dr.
Elizabeth Mahaney & Ms. Dana Castellano, Tampa, Florida.

To contact Dr. Mahaney refer to her web site,
www.SouthTampaTherapy.com or call (813) 240-3237.

Use is limited to printed documents with no lucrative purpose. If you would like

to add your own comments you may do so- just include them in parenthesis with a

note that establishes that the comments are not mine. This information may not be

distributed on a CD or hard disk, or reproduced on another web page, whatever

the nature or purpose.

INTELLECTUAL PROPERTY POLICY

It is our policy to respond to notices of alleged infringement that comply with the

Digital Millennium Copyright Act (the text of which can be found at the U.S.

Copyright Office Web Site, http://LcWeb.Loc.gov/copyright/) and other

applicable intellectual property laws, which may include removing or disabling

access to material claimed to be subject or infringing activity.

EMAIL

We may send out an email to people who have purchased our product(s). We will not give or sell your email address to any third party. You may opt-out of our mailing list at any time. The only effective way to ensure you receive no emails from us is to close your account.

EXTERNAL LINKS

Our site may contain links to other sites. You agree that we do not endorse any other sites and are not liable for any loss or damages related to the content, products or services available through those sites. Further, we are not liable for any damage caused by or resulting from infections from viruses, worms, or Trojan horses, or other malicious computer programs, whether infected from our site or an external link posted on our site. If you have any problems or concerns regarding other sites, please contact their site administrator or webmaster directly.

MISCELLANEOUS

These Terms of Service or Use are governed by and interpreted in accordance with the laws of the state of Florida and the United States, without regard to conflict of law provisions.

These Terms of Service or Use constitute the entire agreement between the parties with respect to the subject matter hereof and supersedes and replaces all prior or contemporaneous understandings or agreements, written or oral, regarding such subject matter. Any waiver of any provisions of the terms of Service or Use will be effective only if in writing and signed by Elizabeth Mahaney.

About The Authors

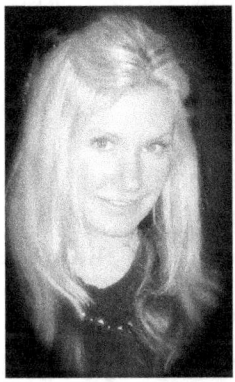

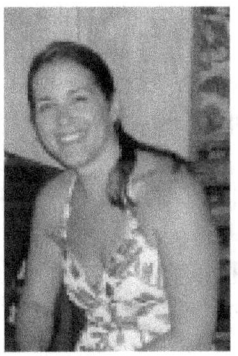

ELIZABETH MAHANEY:
TRAINING AND EXPERIENCE

• Licensed Mental Health Counselor (LMHC) and Marriage and Family Therapist (MFT).

• M.A. Degree in Mental Health Counseling with a concentration and dual enrollment in Marriage and Family Therapy.

• B.A. Degree in Psychology from The University of South Florida.

• Florida Supreme Court Certified Family Law Mediator.

• University of Tampa as a transient student and earned a minor in marketing with concentrations in athletics and personal growth.

• Certified as a Master Neuro-Linguistic Programming Practitioner among other therapeutic applications.

• Ph.D in Clinical Hypnotherapy and affiliated with The National Board of Professional and Ethical Standards.

• National Certified Counselor (NCC).

• Chi Sigma IOTA- Counseling & Academic Honor Society International.

• Board of Director for The Missing Piece of Counseling and Well-Being and The Tampa Bay Association for Women Psychotherapists.

www.SouthTampaTherapy.com

Copyright © 2009,
Dr. Elizabeth Mahaney & Ms. Dana Castellano

DANA CASTELLANO:
TRAINING AND EXPERIENCE

• Clinical Hypnotherapist and affiliated with The National Board of Professional and Ethical Standards.

• Volunteer for The Missing Piece of Counseling and Well-Being Inc. A non-profit organization.

• Neuro-Linguistic Programming Practitioner among other therapeutic applications.

• Over 12 years of Food and Beverage hospitality experience including several healthy, organic menu item contributions.

• Experienced Lifecoach working with several different types of client populations and groups.

www.ingramcontent.com/pod-product-compliance
Lightning Source LLC
Chambersburg PA
CBHW081403280526
45788CB00009B/2968